Sex Games Guide:

Top 21 Hot Sex Games For Bad Girls And Boys

Introduction

Three extraordinary ease alternatives for making a sex amusement for a couple
are:

One of you records on bit of paper the brief points of interest of a sexual dream or
sensual circumstance. At that point that individual needs to carry on what is
composed and the other individual needs to attempt to think about what it is.
When they have speculated effectively, swap turns.

Compose a couple of distinctive sexual exercises on isolated bits of paper. At that
point alternate coaxing them out of a cap - and acting them out!

At the point when sitting in an eatery or bar, watch a portion of the other
individuals around you. Speak together about what you can envision doing to or
with that individual (it might even be another couple). Truly develop your dream
(in spite of the fact that don't talk too uproariously!).

Something else couples ought to recollect about sex games is that they can make
an incredible expansion to sexual foreplay. Particularly for ladies, the more
drawn out the foreplay the better. By presenting one or more games you get the
sexual flames beginning to seethe. Surely attempt to be lively and imaginative
however much as could be expected in your lovemaking. As we said, being perky
was something we all were as youngsters and it is a disgrace that it is something
which grown-ups have lost to an expansive degree. Sex doesn't generally should
be not kidding! Add a couple games to your sex life and it will do a considerable
measure of useful for your relationship when all is said in done.

In case you're short for thoughts for sex games for couples there are various websites offering thoughts. There are even a few games you can buy online or at a grown-up store. Then again, as a rule the best games, much the same as when we were youngsters, are regularly the ones you develop yourself. It doesn't take an excess of creative energy to think of some incredible games. Have a ton of fun!

Chapter 1 – Fun Sex Games For Couples - Time to Add a Twist to Your Relationship

Fun sex games for couples are an awesome wellspring of fuel that will get the flame of your sex life back to a thundering blast. Many people surmise that these games are grimy, unrefined or distorted and don't give them a misgiving. What a disgrace that individuals think along these lines. There are such a large number of distinctive games that are no place close to the universe of unseemly and can give only the energy you are searching for. Playing games is a truly incredible approach to help couples get back in contact with each other and flame up their sex lives.

Presenting fun sex games for couples are an incredible approach to...

- revive the seething powder for your sex life

- build up a much closer and important relationship

- let you and your partner encounter more delight and satisfaction in your relationship

- engage in sexual relations all the more frequently

- hit levels of joy you just imagined about

Regardless of what fun sex games for couples you attempt, recall to utilize your creative energy and truly get into the occasion. Attempt diverse games and figure out which ones you like as well as can be expected, even attempt your hand a making you claim amusement only for you two. Whatever the case, be innovative and realize totally new possibilities. There are such a large number of perspectives to sex that the choices for games are truly perpetual. These games are for you and your partner, not just will you discover them energizing they will likewise bring you two closer than you can envision.

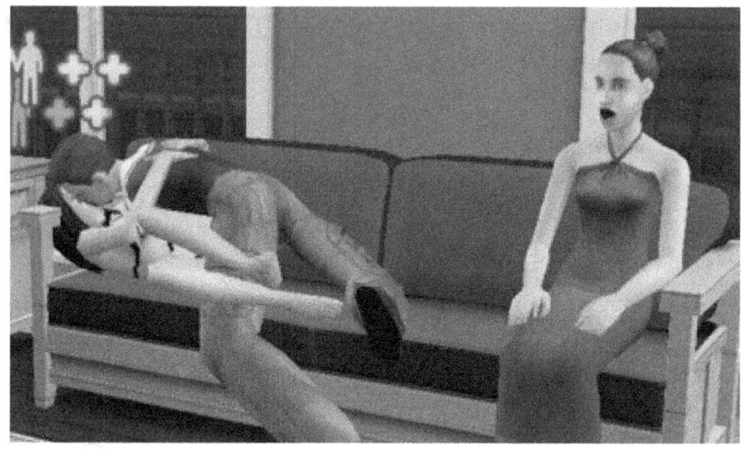

Indeed, even couples with a hot relationship can acknowledge playing games together. Getting a charge out of an amusement as a few considers more creative ability to be utilized to zest things up and allows you to fill a couple dreams. You know they generally say "Couples that play together, stay together!" Below are a couple games you can play at home as a couple for an additional uncommon night.

1.   Truth or Dare - Not just does this amusement permit you to take in a couple of profound dull mysteries about your partner, you additionally get the chance to challenge them to do whatever you need them to do. Nobody can turn down a challenge!

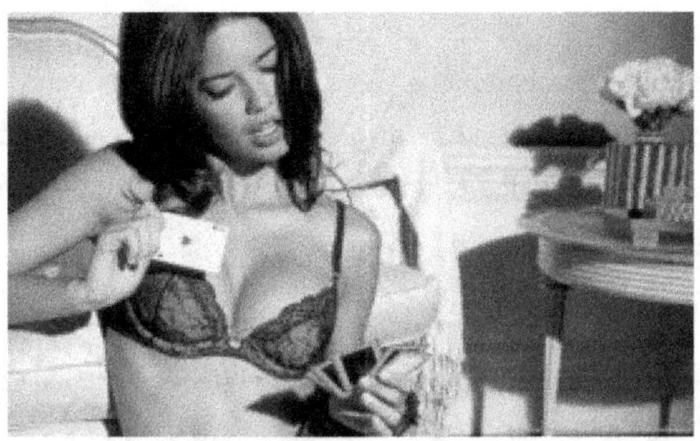

2.   Strip Poker - Actually, it doesn't need to be constrained to simply poker. Any diversion can be changed a bit to be a strip amusement! Can't pay for that lodging you arrived on playing Monopoly? Estimate you'll need to take off garments. Poker is a fun and least demanding amusement to play however.

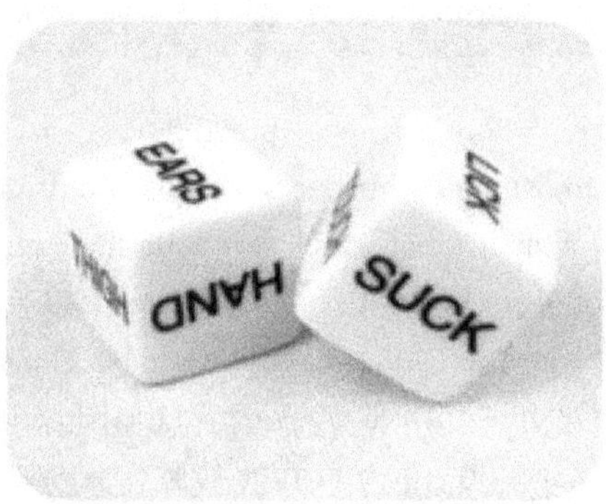

3.   Adult Dice - These exceptional lover's craps have more then quite recently numbers on them! They run from a touch setting out to out and out underhanded, investigating levels of fun loving, sentimental blends. Odds are you won't part one thing two times unnecessarily be that as it may, obviously, it's generally decent If you do!

4.   Sex Game - There are sex games accessible either online or in specific boutiques that are accessible and a mess of good times for any couple to play together. You might need to perform favors, tune in pretending, and so forth. These are dependably amusing to gather in the bag to take with on an excursion as well!

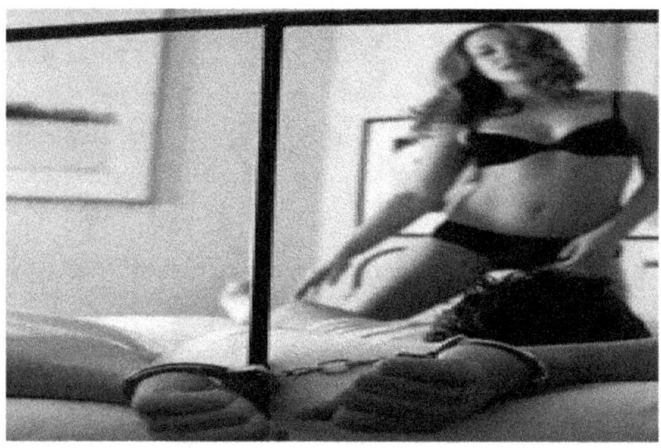

5.   Role Playing - Nothing can beat pretending as a couple. Obviously it's generally enjoyable to astound your partner with an outfit or be unconstrained yet not everybody is actually great with last minute thoughts. You can keep a jug with moved up bits of paper in it with thoughts composed on that you can attract from to choose what your pretending diversion will be. You can make this a week by week diversion or simply draw the majority of the papers with thoughts in one long wild night. It's generally a decent time to keep a couple props helpful like binds for the cop, glasses for the bookkeeper and maybe a sexy French house keeper ensemble as well. The more props and outfits you add to your accumulation, the sultrier your diversion can get to be.

Sex games for couples who have been as one for a considerable length of time, years, and decades, can turn into the ruin of solid relationships, once the general population included come up short on thoughts, and don't know how to reignite the energy in their lives. Different relationships rehash the same lovemaking knowledge again and again, while scanning for an answer that is not found. Both circumstances have created a few relationships to blur away, and have demolished fellowships that ought to have endured forever.

Energy has a tendency to vanish after the "been there, done that" feelings begin to kick in, trailed by snippets of anxiety, weariness, and feeling unsatisfied! An enduring association relies on a few in number parts. How couples identify with one another as companions, not lovers, has vital influence in how their relationship will convey into what's to come. On the other hand, negative sexual pressure because of redundancy, has kept numerous from having a future.

This solid, immediately downloadable digital book comprises of numerous games that are new, simple to get ready and perform, and are not debasing to a relationship. Some of them are as per the following:

- another approach to play with a deck of cards that will prompt astounding peaks.

- an energizing amusement that prompts lovemaking in new places around the home.

- a speculating diversion that prompts blazing craving in ten minutes.

- a diversion that transforms a consistently encounter into 30 minutes of throbbing foreplay.

- an amusement that fortifies bodies in new and energizing ways, while keeping partners asking for additional.

- an amusement that uses blindfolds and nourishment.

- 4 rewards and numerous more games that will lead couples to more important, certain, fulfilled, secure, and orgasmic relationships.

Sex games for couples who need to propel their relationships, have at last arrived and will permit their lives to bloom together, far into what's to come!

Chapter 2 – Passionate Bedroom Sex Games

Feeling exhausted with your sex life? Engages in sexual relations turn into a standard issue? Might you be able to discover just the same old thing new in your partner? May be it's opportunity both of you enjoy some energetic room sex games. These games are certain to transform your ordinary sex life into something extraordinary and your partner will appear like the individual you began to look all starry eyed at interestingly.

Enthusiastic games of sex separation the fatigue of room, as well as open up the correspondence handle and give you motivation to grow your sexual range also. The accompanying games that are talked about beneath will offer you some assistance with unlocking the entryway to a radical new significance of energy.

Underhanded Dice Game is one such amusement in which you allocate an extraordinary intending to every number of ivories. For instance, 1 is for foot knead, 2 is for strip move, et cetera. Every time you toss the shakers, your partner needs to perform the demonstration.

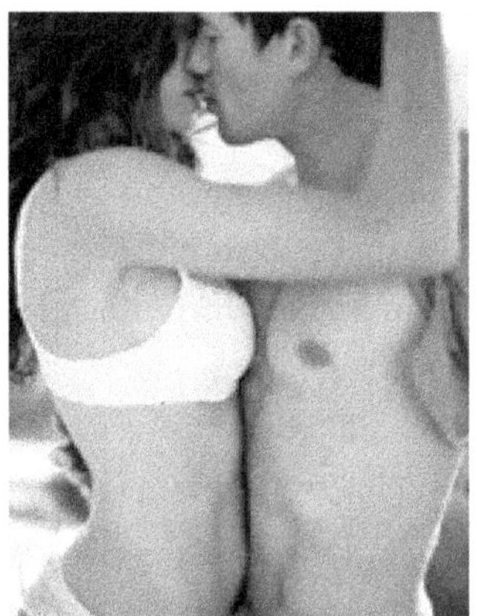

Twist the Bottle is another diversion that proves to be useful at the majority of the times. You presumably recollect that it from your school days. Restore the diversion. The main contrast now is that the stakes are distinctive. The solicitations ought to say - kiss, striptease, and so forth. It's an awesome transform on once you get into the depression. Wardrobe Love can likewise be an extraordinary turn on. Simply cover up in her storeroom and when she touches base to change, shock her with an energetic kiss and some hot foreplay.

You can likewise make great utilization of pretending sex games, as where one partner turns into the shrewd specialist and alternate assumes the part of a patient. This is an energizing and cheerful approach to toss some sizzle in your sex life. You can play out this diversion in distinctive courses, contingent upon how far your creative energy runs wild. As a matter of first importance, decide the part that you and your partner will play. Numerous folks want to assume the part of the insidious specialist against their lover's "powerless" patient. You ought to additionally figure out whether you require ensembles or not. The initial step of this energetic room sex diversion starts with the specialist's examination of his/ her patient. The specialist ought to analyze the bare or half-dressed patient in a nonsexual, proficient manner. On the other hand, after the specialist finds an injury in an erogenous zone (the crotch, the bosoms, posterior or inward thigh, for instance), he/she ought to treat the area tenderly until enthusiasm expends him/her. You have to utilize this pretending situation in a casual way and set aside your opportunity to develop sexual energy. Attempt to utilize dialog as foreplay and continue talking while you are caught up with having intercourse. This will clearly flavor up your love life.

There are huge amounts of fun sex games that you can experiment with your lover to make your night all the more energizing and energetic. Sex games in the room can assist the both of you to get into the right temperament for draw out foreplay, which will bring about hazardous sex later on.

Give me a chance to simply with you 3 fascinating sex games that you can experiment with your lover today evening time:

1.   The Bitchy Nurse. The lady will put on white undies, bras, and leggings, and tackle the part of a medical caretaker in a center. She will get the man to get ready for wellbeing examination. The both of you must get into the parts by being totally clinical. The lady can stroke her lover's masculinity and say that it is to guarantee that it is working fine. At that point the lady ought to make the diversion all the more telling so as to energize the man that she needs to gather semen tests. The both of you can then get into the ride and with the man "giving" her with the semen toward the end of the night.

2. The Chauffeur. The lady will be in control in this amusement, and request that the man be her escort. The "driver" will then drive her to a sex shop where she will go down and purchase a wicked toy. Once in the auto, the lady ought not tell

the man what she has gotten. Keep it a mystery at any rate until after supper. At that point show the toy to him from the rearward sitting arrangement. When he is truly energized, get him to the rearward sitting arrangement and shag the night out with you.

3. The Body Painter. One of you can go about as a painter where you sit your lover down and paint his or her body. Get bare and you make a magnum opus on his or her body. This is an exceptionally sexy act when you touch the territories that are sensual and touchy to your lover. Before you get into this diversion, make sure to see whether your lover has any sensitivities.

Feeling exhausted with your sex life? Has intercourse turned into a standard issue? Would you be able to discover just the same old thing new in your partner? May be it's opportunity both of you enjoy some energetic room sex games. These games are certain to transform your ordinary sex life into something extraordinary and your partner will appear like the individual you became hopelessly enamored with interestingly.

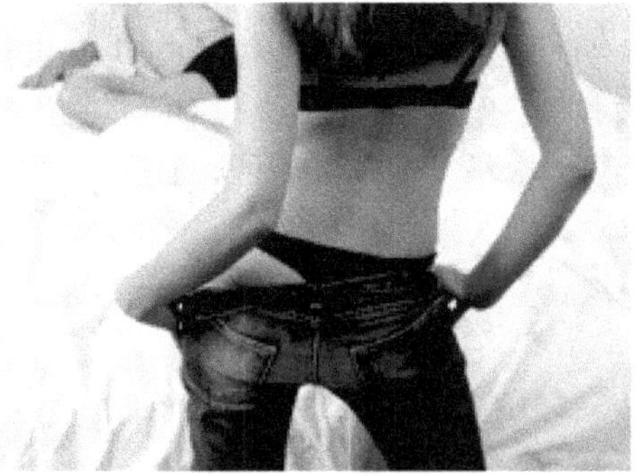

Enthusiastic games of sex separation the fatigue of room, as well as open up the correspondence handle and give you motivation to extend your sexual array also.

The accompanying games that are examined beneath will offer you some assistance with unlocking the entryway to a radical new significance of enthusiasm.

Underhanded Dice Game is one such diversion in which you allocate an exceptional intending to every number of craps. For instance, 1 is for foot rub, 2 is for strip move, et cetera. Every time you toss the shakers, your partner needs to perform the demonstration.

Twist the Bottle is another diversion that proves to be useful at a large portion of the times. You likely recall that it from your school days. Resuscitate the diversion. The main contrast now is that the stakes are distinctive. The solicitations ought to say - kiss, striptease, and so forth. It's an awesome transform on once you get into the section. Storage room Love can likewise be an incredible turn on. Simply stow away in her storeroom and when she touches base to change, astonish her with an energetic kiss and some hot foreplay.

You can likewise make great utilization of pretending sex games, as where one partner turns into the insidious specialist and alternate assumes the part of a patient. This is an energizing and happy approach to toss some sizzle in your sex life. You can play out this diversion in distinctive routes, contingent upon how far your creative energy runs wild. Above all else, decide the part that you and your partner will play. Numerous folks like to assume the part of the devious specialist against their lover's "defenseless" patient.

You ought to likewise figure out whether you require outfits or not. The initial step of this enthusiastic room sex amusement starts with the specialist's examination of his/her patient. The specialist ought to analyze the exposed or half-dressed patient in a nonsexual, proficient manner. Notwithstanding, after the specialist finds an injury in an erogenous zone (the crotch, the bosoms, bum or inward thigh, for instance), he/she ought to treat the district tenderly until energy devours him/her. You have to utilize this pretending situation in a casual way and set aside your opportunity to develop sexual energy. Attempt to utilize dialog as foreplay and continue talking while you are caught up with having intercourse. This will without a doubt zest up your love life.

Chapter 3 – 4 Hot Sex Games For Married Couples

If you've been hitched for any period of time and sex has gotten somewhat stale, don't be too hard on yourself. It's regular for sex to frequently fall by the wayside in a marriage and turn out to be to some degree schedule.

After some time, sex drive decreases, you have less and less time alone together and the time you do have in bed turns out to be to some degree mechanical or unsurprising.

Like I said, don't be too hard on yourself - it happens. Be that as it may, in light of the fact that it happens, doesn't make it right. You and your companion have a commitment to one another to keep your sex life alluring and new. This article is going to demonstrate to you precisely best practices to do that with some smoking hot sex games to shake up your time together and make them shag.

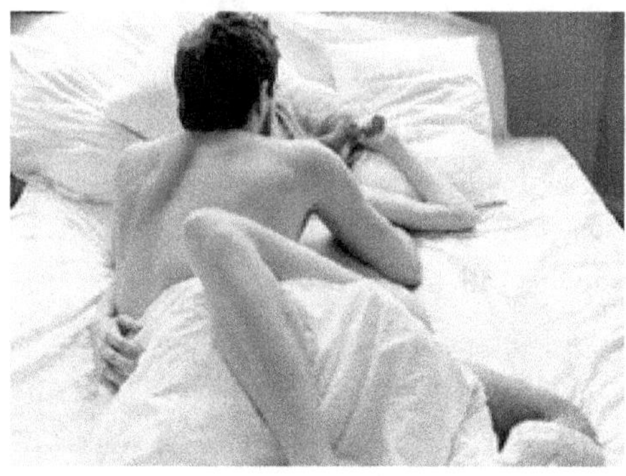

Here are a couple sex games for wedded couples:

• Truth or Dare: A most loved diversion in adolescent gatherings throughout the years, this can be modified to oblige your sexual needs. You and your partner start by composing five mischievous dares on paper pieces and putting them in a dish. Next, you ask your partner "Truth or Dare?" If the answer is Truth, then ask the sexy inquiry you have dependably covertly wanted to inquire. If your partner doesn't reply, then they need to pick one of your Dares. This diversion can be an exceptionally private and in addition learning sexual experience for couples.

• Role playing: This audacious sex diversion is about transforming your sexual dreams into substances. It is possible that you can start by discussing your sexual dreams that you might want to play or you could totally surprise your partner by sprucing up in one of the dream characters. You could be a sexy attendant, a team promoter, a strip artist or any other person you think will turn your partner on. You will require a coordinating suggestive dress to match with the part you are going to play. You then go ahead to play the sexy scenes with your partner. There are unlimited potential outcomes in this sex diversion and this is the reason it is favored by a considerable measure of wedded couples.

• Strip Poker: This is one of the most straightforward approaches to have a great deal of exceptional fun. Both of the partner's start by wearing same number of garments. Every time one of you loses a hand, they need to uproot one of their garments. After one or both of you are exposed, you can continue to request sexual demonstrations of your decision every time you win. If, you are not huge poker fan, you can do this with any card amusement.

• Buy sex games: There are various sex games that can be acquired to reignite your sex life. They run from straightforward prepackaged games to expand sex games with hardware. Actually, hunting and shopping down these games can likewise be a fun experience If you both do it together in the security of your room. Set aside time to investigate all sort of sex games that are accessible for buy online. Appreciate perusing their depiction and examine potential outcomes. You might likewise get a considerable measure of thoughts to imagine your own particular games from them.

Chapter 4 – Naughty Dirty Games to Play With Your Boyfriend Over Text

Nothing can make your sweetheart foresee sex more than filthy games over content. The magnificence of these games is that you are allowed to express whatever you feel as there are no set principles. They likewise introduce the ideal stage to express your dirtiest emotions which you'd experience considerable difficulties to your beau eye to eye.

Grimy games take the craft of temptation and sentiment to the following level which fundamentally makes the relationship additionally energizing. They are moderately simple to start and at the peak of every amusement, your beau wouldn't see any problems with making out with you whenever you meet.

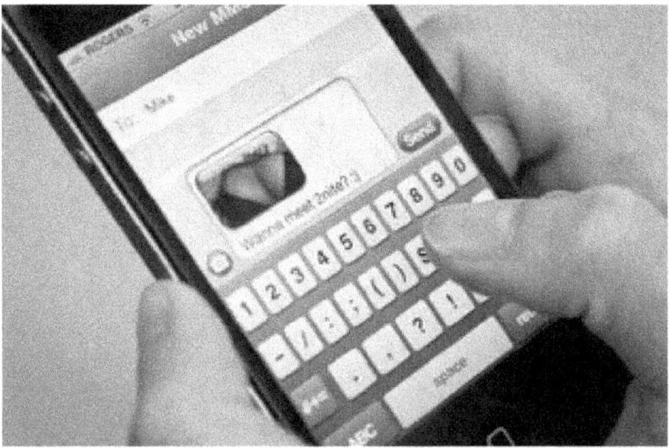

Here are five games you can play;

The shrewd inquiries amusement... This one like the name proposes includes a trade of hot, hot messages all trying to get answers to some insidious inquiries. To play this amusement and achieve the expected objective, begin on a pure note and keep the force going as the diversion heightens. The amusement fundamentally includes asking your beau what he needs and you answer him naughtily. As the diversion advances he will join in and begin putting forth grimy inquiries. The amusement gets to be more blazing as the inquiries get naughtier.

The sexting diversion... This is pretty much like engaging in sexual relations via telephone, yet through instant messages. It includes making a love scene and looking at engaging in sexual relations with your man. The most straightforward approach to begin this is to ask your sweetheart what he is doing. Continue to let him know that you're sleeping and inquire as to whether he needs to go along with you. Obviously he needs to. Get more sexual as he reacts to a state of making him touch himself on the flip side, which is essentially the purpose of the diversion.

The challenging diversion... This is one of the grimy games to play with your beau that is sure to turn both of you on when you're set playing. It includes challenging your partner to answer an irregular mischievous question or requesting that they demonstration it out. With the approach of Smartphones, it's best played by trading devious pictures. Envision challenging your sweetheart to share a photo of his erect penis. He can likewise challenge you to send a photograph of your bosoms et cetera. While this amusement can be hot, bear in mind to erase the photos once you're through playing the diversion.

The round of admission... Let's face honest, all have been through different sexual experiences in our lives; some great, some not very great. The admission diversion includes uncovering the most profound kept sexual privileged insights. Try not to consider the admission amusement excessively important; after all it's only a diversion.

Solicit your man what are some from the most humiliating sexual experiences he's had, how his first sensual caress felt, how it was similar to lick he sweetheart's bosoms and such sorts of stuff. So that the diversion doesn't appear to harp on his past relationships no one but, you can ask him how it feels to be sleeping with you, his most loved positions and the best sexual experience he's ever had with you.

Playing insidious and messy games with your beau is the better approach to tease. It gives you a chance to dive somewhere down into one another's sexual yearnings and in the process brings you closer sexually. These messy games will get him into a sexual state of mind in the blink of an eye. The more you play them, the more you warm up to making out on the following date.

Grimy messaging your partner before you physically meet him later in the day is an impeccable approach to make sexual anticipation. When you send him messages that are gone for making extremely distinct photos of your stripped body you can make certain that he will be brimming with craving whenever he looks at you. Here are a few illustrations of messy messaging that you can send him at this time! Utilize these filthy talk lines on him today evening time!

Chapter 5 – Sex Games With Eyes

For him:

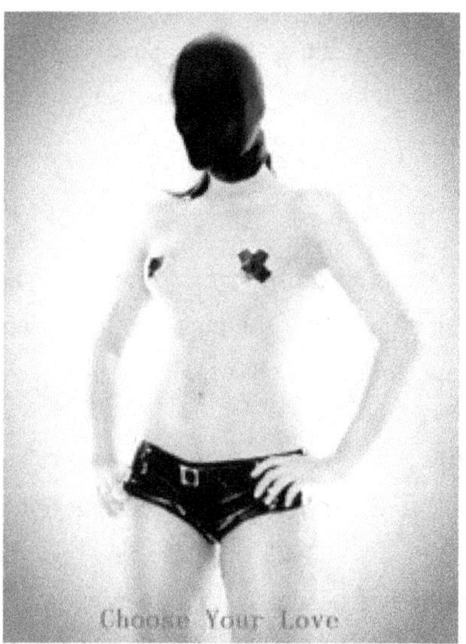

To give you a reasonable cautioning ahead of time, this is likely going to be a standout amongst the costliest temptation thoughts that you'll run over. Be that as it may, as you'll see, it can pay off for quite a long time and years to come.

Advise your woman you might want to take her out to supper - a rich supper that will be loaded with amazements and some extremely unique endowments. There is this one catch, however. She ought to dress pleasantly - her most loved suit, or a sharp coat and skirt - however she is to wear literally nothing underneath.

She'll be blazing with interest yet unquestionably energized. Furthermore, soon she'll be reddening, in light of the fact that you're going to persuade her to give you a look at her concealed fortunes... right in the eatery.

Be enchanting, yet don't be hesitant to ask. She'll look at the space to ensure nobody is looking, and she'll hold up until the server vanishes, yet then she'll give her a chance to pullover fall open just so...

As of right now you'll grin and murmur profoundly. Advise her how lovely and suggestive she is and that you think she merits a prize. Venture into your pocket and haul out one striking gold stud.

Also, that is the means by which the amusement is played. Next, persuade her to give you a chance to touch her - That's privilege, you're going to slide your fingers into her shirt and stroke her bosom in this open spot, and nobody is going to catch on.

Incline close; snatch her lapel as though you're analyzing the fabric, however neglect your hand inside the coat, and inside her shirt. Tenderly brush the back of your hand over her areola. Feel it harden as you move it between your fingers (and watch her battle to keep a straight face). Goodness yes, she's earned another prize. Time to deliver the other stud.

The sheer scrumptious mischievousness of this open enticement might have you both pawing the ground and prepared to skip dessert. There is, on the other hand, one last step - she needs to gain the last bit of gems in your pocket, and at this point she's made sense of how. She'll squirm in her seat, she'll fold her legs, she'll pull at her skirt - and for no less than one brief minute you'll get a look of Paradise.

Try not to be amazed if the new gold chain in your pocket isn't the main thing that is shimmering in the candlelight. When supper - and your private show - is over, head for home.

Furthermore, later on, when she puts on her "unique" gems, look for a grin all over. You may be going to see your little speculation pay off once more... what's more, once more... what's more, once more... what's more, once more.

In today's diversion, you are going to begin by making her insane... at that point you will continue to drive her totally nuts. (Positively, obviously)

On Monday, move your kitchen or lounge seat to the room and place it up against the divider. Try not to say a word in regards to it. Simply abandon it there.

She may move it back, so on Tuesday set it back in the room with a note on it that says, "Don't Touch This!" This would regularly excite her interest just without anyone else's input, however you are going to take it to the placing so as to follow level on it a couple of her sexiest shoes... you know, the ones she wears when she needs to look super-hot... alongside a delightfully "Little Sum'n" blessing only for her.

If she wasn't at that point inquisitive, she'll be climbing the dividers at this moment.

On Wednesday, include a couple of leggings and a fastener belt. Thursday, a sexy skirt. Friday, a shirt. (See how there was no notice of incorporating underwear in the outfit... more on that later)

At this point, she's withering to realize what you have arranged out. She will get some information about it, also. Be that as it may, you're not letting out the slightest peep. (You better not. Stay solid.)

Saturday is at last here. So request that her put it all on. She's presumably going to believe that you're taking her for an extraordinary night out, yet the genuine story is - you're going to have a fabulous time - well, you're going to have a LOT of fun - with her G-Spot... furthermore, that basic seat is going to offer you some assistance with doing it.

An imperative piece of making this work to its most extreme excitement potential, you must be exceptionally agreeable in the main and predominant position. Try not to utilize an excess of words, however say your words with energetic power. Also, when it's the ideal opportunity for you to do your part, own it.

As per... um... unmistakable specialists, there are two interesting positions that are perfect for invigorating the G-Spot. Also, you, you fortunate fallen angel you, are going to do all the empowering... with your penis!

Advise her to sit. Climb up her skirt and open her thighs as you move in for a heavenly kiss. Mess around with it. There's no surge today.

Be that as it may, after you've excited her... what's more, tasted her, and caressed her, and played with her... advise her it's an ideal opportunity to uncover the mystery of the seat.

Advise her to stand up and face it, legs separated yet straight, and twist around sufficiently only to put her hands on the seat for backing. If she didn't feel shrewd some time recently, she certainly does now. Presently, there she is... legs totally open with nothing on under her skirt.

So it's your swing to do what you're there to do... Time for you to sparkle. Slide inside, and ride moderate and simple while the steam begins to assemble.

Presently have her stoop on the seat, laying her arms on the back of the seat. In this radiant position, the leader of your penis is riding over her G-spot with each, single stroke. Try not to let whatever is left of her body get desolate, however.

Stretch around and back rub her clitoris. Cup her bosoms and move her areolas through your fingers. Sink your teeth into her neck and nibble her delicate yet hard. Snack on her ear projection. Be that as it may, above all... continue stroking. Try not to set out stop.

Her whole body - and certainly her G-Spot - will be in this way, amazingly animated that not long after, she'll have an extremely serious, and effective climax.

And all on account of a seat.

Presently every time you have visitors over and somebody sits in it, she'll get all jazzed and giggly.

Pleasantly done.

For her: Different ideas

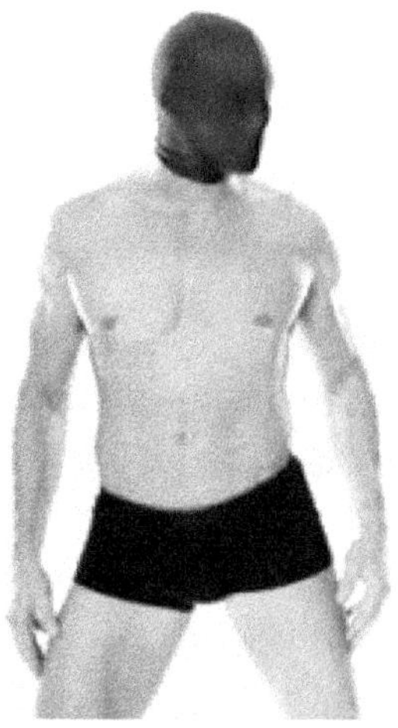

There's no denying that there is a sure vitality to nature that can be portrayed as mysterious. All that daylight and natural air. The fragrance of the trees soggy with the dew noticeable all around. The different sounds and clamors that are originating from every one of the animals in the shrubberies and the trees.

It's animating. It's fortifying. What's more, it's a totally incredible spot for sex. Obviously, no endeavor into the wild is finished without a bottle.

Discover one and put it on the dashboard of his auto with a note... "We should go for a long walk. Somewhere where we can think about the winged animals. What's more, the honey bees."

Obviously, you don't generally require wild. A vast stop or safeguard with loads of trees and praises will do. If it's sufficiently enormous to have strolling trails, then there's a really decent risk that it's sufficiently huge to locate a little protection. In any case, discovering a private and remote alcove is just a large portion of the fight.

Your clothing can be the contrast between an awesome sexual experience or a totally crappy one. The key is to dress for simple access. A long, streaming skirt and a free secure pullover would in all probability do the trap. Also, obviously, no underwear.

Once out on your trek, keep your eyes open for a covered spot out of the way. The best places will presumably be tough - huge rocks, shades and little chasms will offer security from prying eyes underneath. (Unless you need to be seen. Which is a totally diverse story)

Toss out a sweeping and appreciate the landscape. Cooperative with nature. Take in the sights. If you don't see any wild creatures immediately, don't fuss. You'll simply need to make one of your own. A couple of hot kisses and a couple of tight secures will draw out the mammoth in him. If that doesn't transform him into a raving crazy person prepared to rip your garments off, all it takes is a couple of shrewd words whispered in his ear.

Also, once he's all worked up... It's a great opportunity to exploit your closet.

Sit on his thighs and spread your skirt out wide. welcome him to slip his hands underneath. As his fingertips investigate, he will see that there is no clothing. Presently this may end up being some outing all things considered...

Your skirt covers his zipper, and the length of his hands are down there, he should open it up and whip it out. In this way, request that he do only that.

When it's free, run your fingertips along the length of his timber. Stroke his erection through your dress. Draw the fabric over the rigid skin of his firm substance; wrap it up and crush it tight.

It's an effectively suggestive scene. Consider it... he's by and large sexually overhauled by an exceedingly stirred lady, in a spot where other individuals may stop by, and If they did - they wouldn't see a thing.

When you open a couple catches on your pullover, no one but he can glimpse inside. When you slip him in and rapidly, all of a sudden sit on his penis - your free attire covers all. For whatever length of time that you remain focused you can truly make the earth move without being seen. Without a doubt, the length of you don't make any super clear moves that appear as though you're on top riding him.

Presently being heard is another matter. The crackling of sticks and foliage is one thing. The light groaning originating from you is something else. Furthermore, the boisterous howling of your mate when drawing closer peak will be the one to finish it all off.

A "fast in and out" can make starts fly in any relationship. Talking from a man's perspective, there is something to a great degree hot and sexy about climbing up her skirt and getting straight to it.

No foreplay. No sentiment. No bed. Simply crude, hot, wet sex.

It actually works in each relationship. Presently, what about adding a few unconstrained fervors to yours? This week, you're going to surprise your man totally.

Obviously, before you can blink him, you must catch him, and that is the place the genuine fun of this temptation lies. You're going to do it the old style Western path - with a rope. Also, you're going to motivate him to make it for you.

Right on time in the week, let him know you require some rope for an uncommon undertaking you have at the top of the priority list. Not very thick, and around ten feet long. "You wouldn't fret lifting some up for me, will your nectar? You know how I loathe those handyman shops. If you don't mind.

At the point when Saturday moves around, request that he make a tether - and don't stress if his Boy Scout abilities are somewhat corroded. A major tied circle toward the end of the line will do fine and dandy. Much to his dismay, that he's helping you secure his "destruction". When he works it out, say thanks to him and take it from him... and afterward hurl it over him.

You just reserved yourself a major stallion, and now you get the chance to ride them, cowgirl! Drag him over to the stairs and make him sit.

"See this?" Lift your skirt. You have no undies on.

"See this?" Show him a cake clock. Set it to five minutes.

"That is all the time we have, cattle rustler."

Jump on top, and straddle his face. Give him a chance to have a snappy taste of your nectar - there's not any more intense sexual enhancer on the planet, and I'll wager you can practically hear a "pop" as his penis in a flash springs to full consideration.

Pull his trousers down; spread your legs and maneuver him into you. The power of the circumstance will bring about both of you to be touchier than normal. You'll get wetter than you would ordinarily, he'll be harder than he gets regularly. Regardless of the possibility that you move gradually with no genuine revolving, he'll get the opportunity to peak prepared in a matter of a couple of minutes.

What's more, when the clock sounds off - stop!

Sorry yet that is the guideline today. Also, the principles are critical and must not be broken.

If a climax doesn't happen inside of that time limit, well, you can wager he'll be worked up for whatever is left of the day. What's more, you likely won't need to sit tight until night for help.

There will be such a great amount of repressed sexual vitality within his body, that he might pursue you the whole day. If you could arrange your little cowhand/cowgirl session on a day that includes you folks setting off to some sort of get-together, and you don't give him a chance to complete, he will be for all intents and purposes adhered to you the entire night.

He will be whispering mischievous little lines in your ear as you attempt to keep a straight face. He will send you grimy instant messages while you're conversing with other individuals at the gathering - boasting about all the unusual things he's going to do to you when you return home.

His psyche will be so possessed with dreams that it will appear as though he is disregarding others at the gathering. In any case, he's most likely simply going to be considering how he can rope you in, and reset the clock.

Conclusion

Play sex games and truly flavor it up! There are a wide range of sex games to play, games that emphasis on sentiment and closeness, games that attention on foreplay and pretending games are only a couple of the sex games that individuals play.

Sex games can transform a manageable affair into a wild one, or bring you and your partner closer through more cozy encounters. Here are a couple reasons individuals play sex games:

- to expand enthusiasm, when things truly get hot fan the flames of craving,

- for oddity, for example, when we change the area or the season of day, our brains like new encounters,

- to assemble self-regard and certainty, when you feel awesome about who you are and in your body you will ooze sex offer,

- the impression of touch, exotic touch empowers endorphins, what an extraordinary approach to feel great, no big surprise everybody needs the human touch,

- for consistency, standard sex keeps us feeling great,

- to draw in inwardly, sex without an enthusiastic association with your partner is similar to being in a desert rather than a lavish patio nursery.

There are numerous basic games you can play. A basic amusement, for example, perusing Forum Magazine or other sexually unequivocal material with your partner and after that showcasing a most loved entry can bring about bizarrely hot sex play.

Another amusement you can is to follow "Penis" on your lover's back while their eyes are shut. Your lover must obviously think about what word you are following on their back. Zest the amusement up - if your lover can think about what you have followed on the first attempt then you have lost, and must do whatever your lover needs you to accomplish for the following hour. If you should continue following the same word on your lover's back, then they lose, and they should do whatever you need them to accomplish for the following hour.

A sex tabletop game or round of shakers can be enjoyable to play and open up new vistas for you. One such dice amusement is Willy Play. Willy Play gives foreplay proposals for his willy! One bite the dust says things like: suck, snack, stroke and alternate records parts of his willy. Whether you be male or female, straight or gay, some portion of a couple or single, envision what you could do with a couple of shakers like that!

Another sentimental foreplay diversion is the Fleur D'Amour, or blossom of love. This is a solitary red rose that you can present to your lover with a twist. On every petal of this tall-stemmed rose is printed a sexy proposal for lovers to perform on one another. To play you take it in swings to crease back a petal and showcase the proposal, be it a delicate neck rub, a touch of vital tickling, or something more scandalous. When you are done with the diversion you will have no doubt shed the majority of your garments and also your hindrances. The petals of the rose will twist over into spot once you are done, so you can utilize the Fleur D'Amour over and over.

There are huge amounts of different games you can play. If you are keen on discovering sex games do a pursuit on the Internet. There are such a large number of games to browse, you may have a troublesome time selecting.